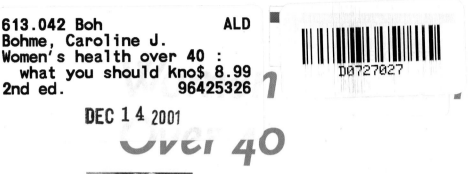

Over 40

what you should know

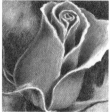

Blackwell
Science

Women's Health Over 40

what you should know

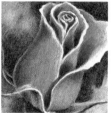

Written by Caroline J. Böhme, MD, FACOG,
Janette Gosch-Weisbrodt, MEd,
and Rona B. Wharton, MEd, RD, LD
Illustrated by Laura L. Seeley

©2001 by Robertson & Fisher Publishing Company. Second Edition.

Written by: Caroline J. Böhme, MD, FACOG; Janette C. Gosch-Weisbrodt, MEd; and
Rona B. Wharton, MEd, RD, LD

Contributing Editors: Karl Bueschenschuetz, DO; Dean J. Kereiakes, MD, FACC; Paul Ribisl, PhD; and
Douglas Wetherill, MS

Illustrated by: Laura L. Seeley

Distributors:
Blackwell Publishing
c/o AIDC
P.O. Box 20, 50 Winter Sport Lane, Williston, VT 05495-0020 USA
(Telephone orders: 800-216-2522; fax orders: 802-864-7626)

Blackwell Science, Ltd.
c/o Marston Book Services, Ltd.
P.O. Box 269, Abingdon, Oxon OX14 4YN, England
(Telephone orders: 44-01235-465500; fax orders: 44-01235-465555)

Printed in Canada
01 02 03 04 5 4 3 2 1 (ISBN:0-632-04537-X)

The Blackwell Science logo is a trademark of Blackwell Science Ltd., registered at the United Kingdom
Trade Marks Registry.

A catalog record for this book is available from the U.S. Library of Congress.

This book is dedicated ...

to all the physicians, staff, and patients who helped me with my training; to my family; and to my best friend and husband Eric.

— Caroline

to my husband Dan, daughter Gretchen, my parents Heinz and Helen, my brother Stuart and family, Stacy and Stephanie, and in loving memory of my sister Susan.

— Janette

to my family, which is much more important to me now that I'm over 40.

— Rona

The authors would like to thank the following people for their input to the second revision of the book: John Young, MD; Angela Ginty; and Paul Neff.

Treatment Disclaimer

This book is for education purposes, not for use in the treatment of medical conditions. It is based on skilled medical opinion as of the date of publication. However, medical science advances and changes rapidly. Furthermore, diagnosis and treatment are often complex and involve more than one disease process or medical issue to determine proper care. If you believe you may have a medical condition described in the book, consult your doctor.

Table of Contents

Introduction

Women's health issues have received growing attention in the past few decades. However, there are 3 conditions which will dominate medical research and treatment in the years to come: breast cancer, osteoporosis, and heart disease.

Women, after age 40, experience an increased risk for each of these diseases. That is why this book focuses on these key topics by explaining risk factors, treatment and — most importantly — prevention.

Reading this book is an important first step in educating yourself and taking an active role in your health and well being. You and your family will benefit from the time you invest taking care of yourself.

— Caroline, Janette, and Rona

Menopause

Pelvic anatomy

Understanding the female anatomy is the first step to understanding what health issues specifically affect a woman. A woman has 2 **ovaries**, 2 **fallopian tubes**, a **uterus**, **cervix**, and **vagina**. The ovary is the storage house for eggs and plays a major role in the production of estrogen. The fallopian tubes are important for the transportation of eggs.

FALLOPIAN
TUBE

UTERUS

OVARY

CERVIX

VAGINA

The uterus has a lining known as the **endometrium**. This lining sheds every month when a woman has a period. It also becomes the womb for pregnancy. The uterus is composed of smooth muscle known as the **myometrium**.

The cervix is the opening to the uterus and is the connection to the vagina. The cervix has an external portion and an internal portion.

Why age 40?

The first menstrual period, known as **menarche**, is a signal that a woman's body is beginning to release eggs. The onset of menses is controlled by many different hormones, including the production of estrogen. A woman will have menstrual cycles approximately 30 to 40 years of her life.

At a certain time in a woman's life, the ovaries are no longer able to produce estrogen. At this time, menstruation ceases. **Menopause** can occur surgically by removal of the ovaries or naturally through aging. The average age for the onset of menopause is 51; it usually occurs sometime between ages 48 and 55.

What happens during menopause?

When menopause occurs naturally, it does not happen overnight. It is a gradual process.

Physical and emotional changes can begin to occur several years before a woman reaches menopause. These changes begin when a woman is in her 40s. This time period is known as **perimenopause**. During perimenopause, a woman may experience mood swings, hot flashes, and a change in the cycles of her period. The menopausal experience is different for each woman.

Post-menopausal concerns

The time after menopause is known as the **post-menopausal** period. Women who are post-menopausal have many health issues to consider.

If women understand the important health issues of menopause at an earlier age, they can make the transition into menopause more easily. Also, by understanding these issues, a woman may be able to identify her risks and possibly prevent disease.

Among the most important health issues for women over 40 to understand are: **breast cancer, osteoporosis,** and **coronary heart disease**.

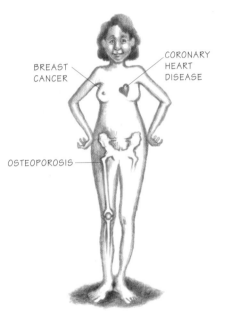

BREAST CANCER

CORONARY HEART DISEASE

OSTEOPOROSIS

Breast Cancer

Anatomy of the breast

Women's ribs are covered with chest muscles. A lining covers these muscles. The breast itself is composed of **fat, lymph vessels, blood vessels**, and the **milk-producing system**. The lymph vessels lead to **lymph nodes** under the arm, above the collarbone, and in the chest. The lymph system is the "fighter" system in our bodies.

LYMPH NODES

FAT

MILK-PRODUCING SYSTEM

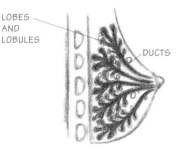

LOBES
AND
LOBULES

DUCTS

Each breast has about 20 sections that are called **lobes**. Each lobe ends in milk-producing glands or **lobules**. Thin tubes called **ducts** connect the lobules to the **nipple** to allow for the passage of milk.

What is cancer?

Our bodies reproduce cells through cell division. Cells go through **cell differentiation**, which determines which cells will perform each specialized function within the body. Life is like a puzzle. The cells in our bodies grow and fit together in a very particular way ...

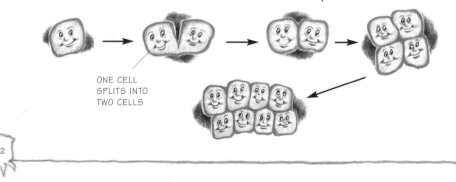

ONE CELL
SPLITS INTO
TWO CELLS

Cancerous cells lack control and pattern. They undergo cell division rapidly without stopping. The result is a crowding of the normal cells. This crowding robs the healthy cells of available nutrients and eventually leads to the death of healthy cells. The puzzle or network of normal cells becomes damaged or interrupted.

CANCER CELL

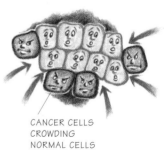

CANCER CELLS
CROWDING
NORMAL CELLS

13

The mass of cancerous cells becomes a tumor. These masses can continue to grow and destroy neighboring healthy tissue.

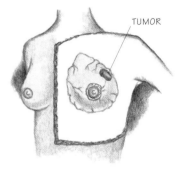

TUMOR

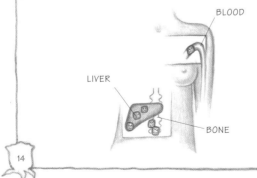

BLOOD

LIVER

BONE

Tumors can also spread, or **metastasize**, to other parts of the body through the blood or lymph system.

Why is screening for cancer so important?

Early detection is the best protection. Cancer may occur in almost any organ of the body, and each type of cancer has its own growth rate. Diagnosis is important to determine the type, location, and extent to which the cancer has spread. The earlier the cancer is diagnosed, the better the woman's chances for survival.

What causes cancer?

Cancer may be caused by multiple factors. **External** factors include chemicals, radiation, viruses, and the environment. **Internal** factors include hormones, heredity (family history of cancer in a mother or sister), immune system, and metabolic conditions. No single factor explains why cancer growth occurs.

What are the risk factors for breast cancer?

Just because you have one or more of the following risk factors does not mean you will eventually develop breast cancer.
It means you must be especially aware of your body and have routine screenings for breast cancer.

Certain risk factors may increase your chances of developing breast cancer:

- Significant family history, especially mother or sister
- Failure to ovulate or release an egg regularly (irregular periods)
- Age at menopause older than 55
- Obesity, diabetes, high-fat diet
- Never having children
- Having your first child after age 30
- Unusual cells found in a breast lump
- Excessive alcohol consumption
- Early menarche

Signs and symptoms of breast cancer

These include a lump in the breast, discharge from a nipple — especially green or red, change in the shape of one or both breasts, indentation of breast skin or "peau de orange" that resembles dimpling, or redness of breast skin.

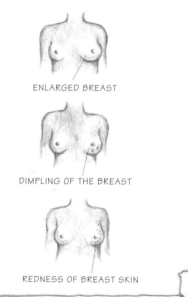

ENLARGED BREAST

DIMPLING OF THE BREAST

REDNESS OF BREAST SKIN

Routine screening for breast cancer is very important. It begins with self-examination starting at age 20. **Every woman should check her breasts monthly**. The best 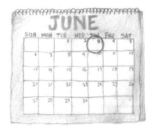 time for this is a week after your period begins. If you no longer menstruate, you should pick the same time every month.

Your doctor should examine your breasts every year.

A breast self-exam is performed using your fingertips. You should start feeling **under your arm** and go around your breast in a circular motion. You should feel from under your collarbone to your breastbone. This should be done on both sides.

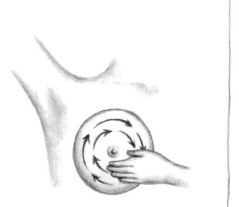

A convenient time to do a self-examination may be when you are taking a shower.

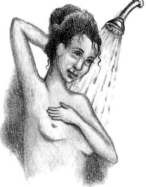

Always look at your breasts in the mirror. You should also squeeze your breasts from the bottom to check for discharge from your nipples. If discharge arises from your nipple, you should contact your doctor.

What if I feel a lump or my doctor feels a lump? Should I assume I have cancer?

No! Just because you feel a lump, do not assume that it is breast cancer. Lumps can be caused by factors other than cancer. An **abscess**, **inflammation**, **clogged duct**, **cyst**, and **fibroadenoma** are some of the **benign** (noncancerous) conditions that may cause lumps in the breast.

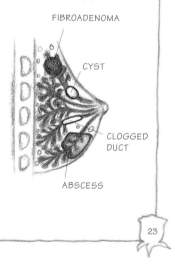

FIBROADENOMA

CYST

CLOGGED DUCT

ABSCESS

All lumps should be reported to your doctor immediately and checked promptly. You may be asked to get a **mammogram**. Additionally, an **ultrasound** may be ordered to determine if the lump is fluid-filled or **cystic**.

ULTRASOUND

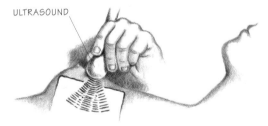

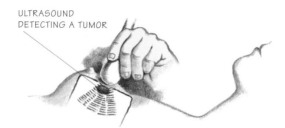

ULTRASOUND
DETECTING A TUMOR

If the lump is only a cyst, the fluid may be removed with a needle and analyzed to determine if it is **malignant** (cancerous). If the lump reappears, if the fluid tested contained malignant cells, or if the lump is not filled with fluid, it may be removed by a method known as a **biopsy**. The biopsy, or lump sample, will also be analyzed for malignancy.

Mammogram

You may not be able to feel a lump smaller than an almond or a pea. This is why a mammogram is so important. It can detect lumps one-tenth of the size that you can feel. A positive mammogram may be a sign, though not proof, that cancer is present.

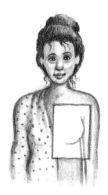

A mammogram is simply an X-ray of your breast. Ordinarily, your first or **baseline** mammogram should be taken between ages 35 and 40 if you have any risk factors. However, it may be done sooner depending on your family history. Unfortunately, mammograms may not be as effective at detecting breast cancer in younger women due to the denseness of the breast tissue.

The current recommendation is to get a mammogram every 1 to 2 years, starting at age 40, and every year after age 50. You should talk to your doctor to see when a mammogram is right for you.

Invasive disease

When cancerous cells spread to nearby or underlying tissue, they are considered **invasive**. Invasive breast cancer is often detected as a lump during a breast exam or as a mass on a mammogram.

Breast cancer staging

Cancers are categorized by a process called **staging**. Doctors determine the **stage** of a cancer according to the tumor size, location, and whether it has spread to other organs or lymph nodes. This can be performed through **examination**, **X-rays**, and/or **surgery**, depending on the type of cancer. The different stages affect the prognosis and treatment of a woman who suffers from cancer.

Breast cancer is generally classified into 4 stages. Stage IV is the most advanced cancer as the cancer has spread to other organs.

Treatment

Two types of treatment are typically chosen for breast cancer:

1) **local treatment** — treatment targeted at a specific site

2) **systemic treatment** — treatment throughout the entire body

Several factors influence the type of treatment chosen. The stage of the disease; the size, type, and location of the tumor; your age and physical health; size of breasts; menopausal status; and results of other laboratory tests are all taken into consideration.

Local treatment

Local treatment includes:
   1) surgery
   2) radiation therapy

Stage I and Stage II cancers may be treated with local treatments. In some cases, these treatments will be combined with systemic treatments.

1. Surgery

Women with breast cancer may undergo one of the following types of surgery:

- **lumpectomy** — removing only the breast lump and some surrounding tissue
- **partial** or **segmental mastectomy** — removing the tumor, surrounding tissue, and chest muscle lining
- **total mastectomy** — removing the breast tissue
- **modified radical mastectomy** — removing the breast tissue, some lymph nodes, and chest muscle lining

- **radical mastectomy** — removing the breast tissue, lymph nodes, chest muscle, and surrounding tissue. This procedure is rare.
- **axillary lymph node dissection** — removing lymph nodes in the axillary region for treatment and/or staging purposes.

Possible side effects of surgery include swelling, loss of strength, stiffness, numbness or tingling, bleeding, infection, and/or blood clots.

2. Radiation therapy

High-energy radiation is concentrated on a particular site in an attempt to destroy or control cancerous cell growth. Radiation can come from a machine (external) or from implanted radioactive material (internal). Radiation treatment for the breast is generally external. Other organs affected with cancer may be treated with internal radiation.

External treatment for the breast may occur on a daily basis for a short period of time. This is typically an outpatient procedure. It is usually done in conjunction with a lumpectomy (see page 33).

Systemic treatment

Systemic treatment, which involves chemotherapy, is typically combined with local treatment for Stage III and Stage IV cancers.

With **chemotherapy**, your doctor will use a combination of drugs that enter the bloodstream via the mouth, vein, or muscle. There are many types of chemotherapy. Treatment is usually performed on an outpatient basis.

Several treatments may be necessary and can be given in cycles:

treatment → recovery,

treatment → recovery, etc.

Possible side effects of chemotherapy include hair loss, nausea, diarrhea, weight loss, dry mouth, and/or infertility.

Oral chemotherapy

SERMS — Selective Estrogen Receptor Modulators — are a class of estrogen-like hormonal medications that have different actions on select tissues. Each medication in this class is somewhat different.

SERMS can affect certain tissues including the breast, bone, and endometrium (lining of the uterus). SERMS are most often used for treatment of breast cancer and osteoporosis.

SERMS can be used to help in the long-term treatment of certain types of breast cancer. Research is also under way to determine what role (if any) SERMS can play in breast cancer prevention.

Side effects of these medications may be similar to menopause, including hot flashes, irregular vaginal bleeding, and vaginal dryness.

Summary

One in 8 women will develop breast cancer. You need to know your risks. You should see your doctor yearly for a breast exam. You also should perform a monthly self-examination. It is very important to work with your doctor to determine what screening is best for you. If you have breast cancer, it is vital to know your treatment options. There are many new treatments on the horizon, so you should consult with your doctor.

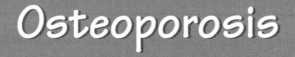

Bones

Our bodies are made up of 206 bones which form our skeletons. Bones provide the structural support for our bodies and protect vital organs.

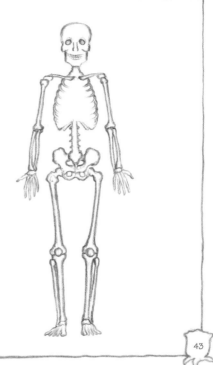

Bones are a complex organization of tissues. They are formed from a mesh-like structure which includes **collagen fibers, calcium, phosphate, fluoride, minerals,** and **water.** These materials combine to produce a structure (bone) that is extremely strong while at the same time somewhat flexible.

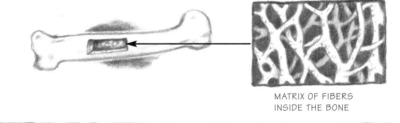

MATRIX OF FIBERS
INSIDE THE BONE

In addition to providing structure and support, our bones also serve as a kind of **"bank"** for minerals used by the body. Bones hold the majority of the body's calcium supply (about 99%). Calcium is also found in the **muscle cells, blood,** and the **lymph system**. Calcium is necessary to perform several functions including maintaining our heartbeat (muscle contraction) and maintaining normal blood pressure.

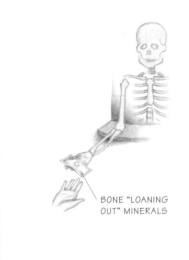
BONE "LOANING OUT" MINERALS

If there is not enough calcium in the blood to perform these bodily functions, calcium will be released from the bones to correct this deficiency in the blood. This process is known as **resorption**. Bones may be broken down to **"loan out"** minerals.

OSTEOCLAST

When resorption occurs, construction-worker-type cells called **osteoclasts** break apart some of the bone.

Resorption is like a jackhammer breaking apart a sidewalk. When the bone breaks apart, it enables needed minerals (**calcium** and **phosphate**) to go into the bloodstream.

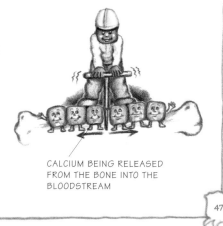

CALCIUM BEING RELEASED FROM THE BONE INTO THE BLOODSTREAM

However, the body needs to replace bone lost due to resorption. To do this, the bone cells take up calcium from the digestive tract to use as building blocks to make new bone. This

CALCIUM BEING ABSORBED BY THE BODY

process is called **formation**. To rebuild bone, the bone cells must have extra calcium available to them from the foods you eat. Calcium is available from many foods. Milk and other dairy products are excellent sources of calcium.

Calcium absorbed from the diet may be used to help build new bone cells. **Osteoblasts** are the "bone-building cells."

OSTEOBLAST

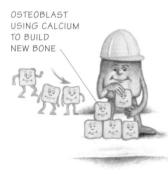

OSTEOBLAST USING CALCIUM TO BUILD NEW BONE

Osteoblasts use calcium to build new **bone cells. Formation** not only helps replace the calcium supply, it also keeps the bones "renewed" by replenishing tissue and bone density.

Osteoporosis

Osteoporosis is a disease in which the bones become fragile and may eventually break. Osteoporosis literally means "porous bones." As we age, **osteoclast activity** (resorption) increases and **osteoblast activity** (formation) decreases. This causes an imbalance in the bone "renewal" process. When there is not complete formation or replacement of bone, the bone weakens and osteoporosis often occurs.

WEAK BONE

Our bones get stronger as we grow, until we reach **"peak bone mass"** when we are in our late 20s or early 30s. After that time, we gradually lose bone mass. During their lives, women **lose** between **30%** to **40%** of their peak bone mass, and men **lose 20%** to **30%** of their peak bone mass.

With osteoporosis, there is a faster loss of bone mass and, therefore, bone strength. Bones can no longer carry the weight they once could. This can lead to bone fractures, especially in the **hips**, **spine**, and **wrists**. Osteoporosis may decrease your ability to perform daily tasks independently and decrease overall quality of life.

Women are **4 times** more likely than men to suffer from osteoporosis. In fact, **1** in **6** women will suffer from a hip fracture during their lifetimes. Hip fractures may result in complications such as **pneumonia**. As the "Baby Boomers" get older and the geriatric population expands, osteoporosis will become an even bigger concern.

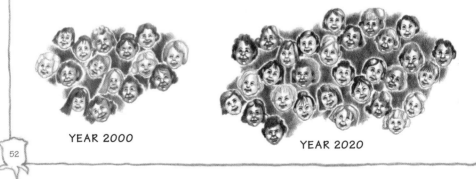

YEAR 2000

YEAR 2020

What is my risk for developing osteoporosis?

Risk factors associated with the onset of osteoporosis include:

- Age 55 or older
- Family history of osteoporosis
- Caucasian or Asian descent
- Women who are thin or small boned
- Women past menopause who have low estrogen levels
- Certain medical conditions or medications

Additional risk factors for osteoporosis include:

- Cigarette smoking
- Excessive consumption of alcohol
- Lack of exercise (primarily weight bearing)
- Too little calcium in the diet
- Early menopause (before age 45)
- Never having children
- Excessive caffeine intake
- Gastric surgery
- Excessive consumption of soft drinks, both caffeinated and caffeine-free

Symptoms

Some common symptoms of osteoporosis include back pain and loss of height. Sometimes there may be no symptoms at all. A classic sign of osteoporosis is a **"dowager's hump,"** or bowing of the upper spine. This is caused by a collapse of the bones of the spine. If you have these or any other symptoms, or if you think you may be at risk for osteoporosis, consult your doctor.

Screening

Screening is an important step in identifying women at risk of developing osteoporosis. The risk factors mentioned earlier can help you and your doctor determine if you need special testing for osteoporosis.

The first step in screening is having your doctor perform an annual history and physical examination. Your doctor can determine if you are at an increased risk for developing osteoporosis and need a **DEXA scan, QCT scan, RA scan,** or other special evaluation. As an example, we will describe one test — the DEXA scan.

Dual energy X-ray absorbitometry (DEXA) scan

DEXA is currently accepted as the most accurate method for diagnosing osteoporosis. The DEXA scan measures bone density and focuses on the density of the spine, the hip, and the wrist. These are the areas at highest risk for fractures in patients with osteoporosis.

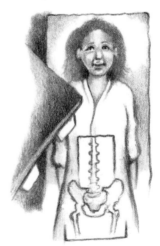

Prevention

You can help to prevent osteoporosis and improve your overall health by modifying your lifestyle:

1) **Do not smoke.**

   Smoking can affect the bone by decreasing bone mass. A woman who smokes has a greater risk of developing osteoporosis. This can increase your risk of fracture, especially in the hip.

2) **Limit alcohol and caffeine consumption.**

   Caffeine and alcohol decrease bone mass. Caffeine also blocks the absorption of calcium by binding to it in the stomach. For this reason, you should wait at least 1 hour after taking a supplement or eating calcium-rich foods before drinking caffeine.

3) Exercise regularly.

Weight-bearing exercise, such as walking, and strength training can actually promote increased bone mass. Exercise also helps to maintain muscle mass and reduce fat mass. Increased strength and flexibility help maintain balance and limit falls that lead to broken bones.

4) Eat healthful foods.

Because each person is very different, it is important that you discuss your diet with your doctor or a registered dietitian. Here are some general recommendations to get you started.

Proper nutrition

Everyone, especially women, must get both **calcium** and **vitamin D** in their diets, either through food sources or through supplementation. The proper amounts of **calcium** may be obtained by eating dairy products, leafy greens, yogurt, nuts, and whole grains.

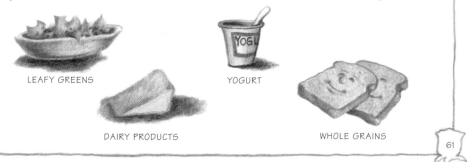

LEAFY GREENS

YOGURT

DAIRY PRODUCTS

WHOLE GRAINS

Vitamin D is needed to absorb calcium into the body. Vitamin D is made when the body absorbs sunlight in skin and combines it with a form of cholesterol. Excessive sun exposure may be harmful, but 30 minutes a day is effective in producing sufficient amounts of vitamin D provided that skin is exposed to natural, outdoor sunlight.

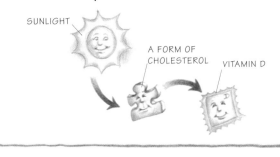

SUNLIGHT

A FORM OF CHOLESTEROL

VITAMIN D

People who live in northern climates of the United States may not achieve adequate sunlight exposure. Contact your doctor to find out if you should take calcium supplements and vitamin D.

Vitamin D can be found in milk and foods like broccoli or salmon. The recommended daily allowance for vitamin D is 400 I.U. An 8-ounce glass of milk contains about 100 I.U. of vitamin D. The vitamin can also be taken as a food supplement.

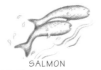
SALMON

BROCCOLI

MILK

Medications for treatment and prevention of osteoporosis

1. Hormone replacement therapy (HRT)

HRT is a combination of **estrogen** and **progesterone**. Estrogen helps reduce the risk of osteoporosis by slowing bone resorption. Progesterone is added to offset some of the effects of estrogen. The earlier HRT is started after menopause, the more beneficial it becomes. Therapy must be used continuously to prevent bone loss. If bone loss has already begun, HRT may still prevent further bone loss (also see pages 139-142).

2. Calcium intake

Calcium absorption is at its peak during the bone-building phase of adolescence. Your ability to absorb calcium decreases slowly. In fact, after age 65, less than 50% of calcium from food and supplements is absorbed.

Calcium is an important part of a woman's nutritional needs. A calcium supplement is usually needed if you do not have **3 to 4 cups** of milk or yogurt each day.

Here are the recommended daily calcium intakes
for a woman during various ages of her life:

- Age 11 through
  age 24   1,200 to 1,500 mg/day
- Pregnancy   1,200 mg/day
- Premenopausal   1,000 mg/day
- Postmenopausal   with HRT* 1,000 mg/day
                                without HRT* 1,500 mg/day

*hormone replacement therapy

Calcium carbonate and **calcium citrate** are two very good forms of calcium supplements. However, not all of the calcium or calcium carbonate may be absorbed completely by the body. Consult your doctor about which supplement is best for you.

3. Bisphosphonates

These medications reduce bone resorption by inhibiting osteoclast activity. They are an effective alternative for women who want to avoid HRT, are not candidates for HRT, or cannot tolerate hormone therapy. Bisphosphonates can be used for treatment and prevention of osteoporosis.

4. Calcitonin

Calcitonin is naturally produced in the body and inhibits bone resorption. Calcitonin is also available as a medication that can be used for treatment of osteoporosis but may be less effective than some other treatments.

5. SERMS (Selective Estrogen Receptor Modulators)

SERMS may also play a role in preventing osteoporosis. Certain SERMS have a positive effect on bone, much like estrogen. SERMS may help increase bone mineral density and are a desirable alternative to HRT because they may not affect breast tissue and the lining of the uterus.

SERMS are also used to treat some types of breast cancer (see pages 39-40).

Again, it is important to talk to your doctor about which treatment is right for you. You should always talk to your doctor about risks, screenings, and treatment options.

Heart Disease

Why discuss heart disease? A 1995 Gallup study revealed that women considered themselves twice as likely to die of breast cancer than from heart disease. In reality, women are **8 times** more likely to die of heart disease than breast cancer.

Heart disease is the leading cause of death for women — more than **all** forms of cancer, diabetes, and lung disease combined.

Prior to menopause, women experience a much lower incidence of heart disease than men of the same age. However, once women reach menopause, they have a much greater incidence of heart disease, and they are less likely than their male counterparts to survive a heart attack.

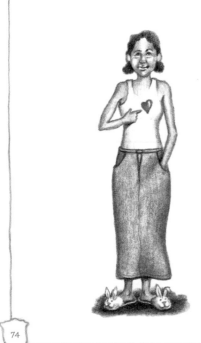

The heart

The heart is a muscle.
It pumps blood to the
head and the body.
It is about the size of
your fist and sits just
to the left of the
middle of your chest.

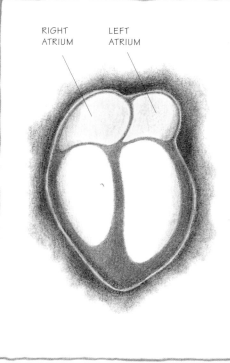

RIGHT ATRIUM

LEFT ATRIUM

The heart is asymmetrical. It is made up of 4 chambers. The top 2 chambers are called the **atria**. The atria collect blood returning to the heart. The atria then dump the blood into the ventricles.

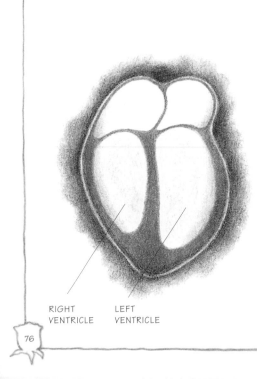

RIGHT
VENTRICLE

LEFT
VENTRICLE

The bottom 2
chambers are called
the **ventricles**. The
ventricles are larger
than the atria, and
the left one is more
muscular. When the
ventricles contract,
they force blood out of
the heart to different
parts of the body.

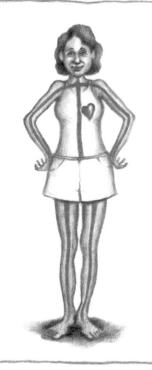

Arteries and veins wind throughout the body carrying blood. Arteries carry blood away from the heart. Veins carry blood back to the heart.

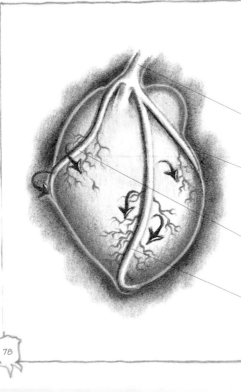

The heart has its own arteries to provide blood to the heart muscle.

The **aorta** supplies blood to the arteries of the heart as well as to the rest of the body.

The **circumflex artery** supplies blood to the lateral or side aspect of the heart.

The **right coronary artery** provides blood to the back or underside of the heart.

The **left anterior descending artery** supplies blood to the front of the heart.

To give you some idea of their size, the **coronary arteries** are only about the size of a strand of spaghetti.

(APPROXIMATE SIZE OF SPAGHETTI)

At birth, the inside of the arteries, including the coronary arteries, is slippery — similar to a nonstick pan. The blood cells (represented by the small cars) flow smoothly through the arteries.

BLOOD FLOW

What happens to an artery during a person's lifetime?

Fatty streaks in the arteries start to develop in the first decade of life as a result of lipids moving into the cell wall of the artery.

LIPIDS MOVING INTO THE ARTERY WALL

These fatty streaks may become more advanced **atherosclerotic lesions** in the presence of risk factors such as smoking, high blood pressure, obesity, high cholesterol, and physical inactivity. The fatty streaks may then progress to **atheromas** and **fibroatheromas**, which are more "advanced lesions" and are often referred to as **plaque**.

ATHEROSCLEROTIC LESION

BLOOD FLOW

Buildups may occur at different points along the length of the artery. Plaque buildups are not limited to the arteries of the heart. They can occur and restrict blood flow in arteries throughout your body.

PLAQUE BUILDUP

The total blockage of the artery may occur due to: a) the **buildup** of plaque, b) the formation of a blood clot on the plaque, or c) the plaque **rupturing** and causing a larger blood clot to form. The complete blockage of the artery is called an **occlusion**.

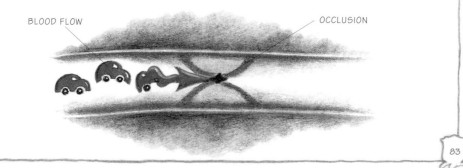

BLOOD FLOW

OCCLUSION

An artery that is completely blocked has no blood flowing through it. If the heart muscle does not receive blood, then it does not receive nutrients and oxygen.

When the heart does not receive oxygen, it experiences **ischemia**. This may result in **heart pain** (angina) or a **heart attack**. Ischemia, if prolonged and severe enough, may cause a portion of the heart muscle to die (heart attack).

What are some symptoms of a possible heart attack?

- **Angina**, or heart pain, usually felt as a pressure, ache, tightness, squeezing, or **burning sensation** under the breastbone and often extending to the neck, jaw, shoulders, or down the arm (most frequently the left arm)
- **Nausea**
- **Shortness of breath** and/or **sweating**

Women may experience fewer symptoms than men.

Quite often, people who are having a heart attack say they feel like "an elephant is standing on my chest."

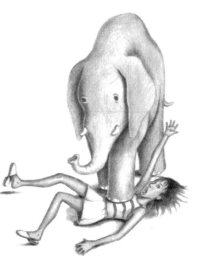

What if you experience heart problems?

What's next?

Your doctor may refer you to a heart specialist called a **cardiologist**. The cardiologist may have to consider several options including **medications** or surgical intervention such as **angioplasty** or **bypass surgery**.

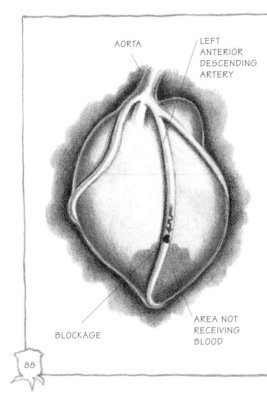

AORTA

LEFT ANTERIOR DESCENDING ARTERY

BLOCKAGE

AREA NOT RECEIVING BLOOD

Suppose there is a sudden blockage (**thrombosis**) in the left anterior descending artery.

The shaded area in the drawing is not receiving blood. If this portion of the heart goes too long without enough oxygen, then the muscle may die.

Thrombolytics

Most often, a heart attack is caused by a **blood clot** (thrombus) at a site of **atherosclerotic plaque disruption** within the coronary artery. Blood clots can completely block blood flow in the artery and cause a heart attack. If a person gets to a hospital emergency room, usually within 30 minutes of the onset of chest pain, a class of medications called **thrombolytics** may be used to dissolve these clots and restore coronary blood flow. The restoration of blood flow to the heart muscle can save heart muscle and reduce the chance of dying. Thrombolytics are most beneficial if given soon after the onset of heart attack symptoms.

Certain individuals may not be candidates to receive thrombolytics, including individuals who have had a recent stroke, surgery, or trauma that would increase the risk of serious bleeding. Likewise, individuals with bleeding peptic ulcers, very high blood pressure, or very advanced age may be at increased risk with thrombolytic therapy. An alternative to thrombolytic therapy for a heart attack is **coronary angioplasty**.

Angioplasty

Angioplasty is a procedure by which the cardiologist inserts a balloon catheter over a thin wire across a blockage of a coronary artery.

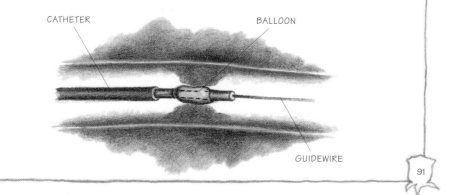

CATHETER

BALLOON

GUIDEWIRE

The balloon is inflated to compress the plaque.
This is repeated as necessary by the cardiologist.

Inflating the catheter compresses and breaks apart the plaque. This allows more room for the blood to flow. The balloon catheter also stretches the elastic wall of the artery. Small tears occur on the inside of the artery wall and slightly injure the artery wall as a result of balloon catheter inflation.

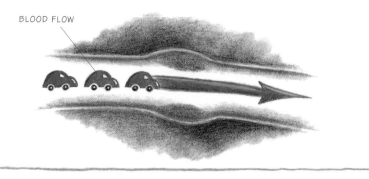

BLOOD FLOW

Unfortunately, these balloon catheter injuries expose substances from inside the atherosclerotic plaque and the artery wall that promote formation of blood clots.

Complications of this procedure may include a heart attack, repeat angioplasty, the need for emergency coronary bypass surgery, and even death.

Stents

In certain instances, the cardiologist may decide to insert a **stent** inside the coronary artery. The stent, usually made of stainless steel, functions as a scaffold to hold open the inside of the coronary artery.

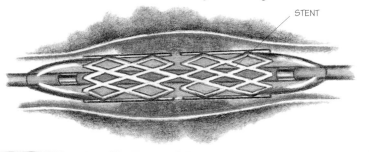

STENT

Stents are usually put in place using a balloon angioplasty catheter. Stents can reduce the incidence of both 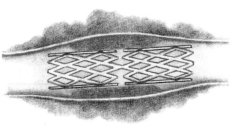 short- and long-term coronary artery reocclusion. Stents can seal and "tack up" tissue flaps within the artery that are created when a balloon catheter injures the artery.

Bypass surgery

Bypass surgery is a cardiovascular procedure designed to correct blood flow to the heart that angioplasty cannot correct. The cardiovascular surgeon uses a piece of artery and/or vein to reroute blood around the blockage.

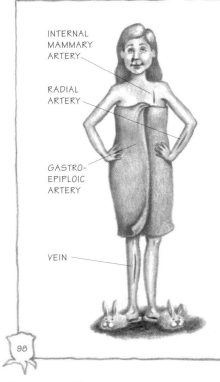

INTERNAL
MAMMARY
ARTERY

RADIAL
ARTERY

GASTRO-
EPIPLOIC
ARTERY

VEIN

The surgeon may use a
vein from the leg, and/or
the internal mammary
artery found in the
chest, and/or the
gastroepiploic artery
of the stomach, and/or
the radial artery of the
forearm.

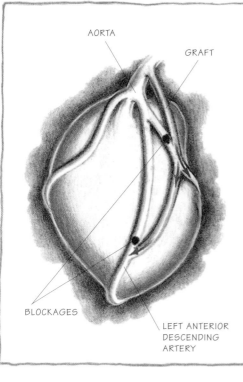

AORTA

GRAFT

BLOCKAGES

LEFT ANTERIOR
DESCENDING
ARTERY

The vein is attached to the aorta. The supply of blood is then rerouted around the blockage. One piece of vein may be used for multiple bypasses. The number of blockages where blood has been rerouted — not the number of veins used — determines the number of bypasses.

If the internal mammary artery is used, the artery originates from a branch off the aorta and is attached directly below the blockage.

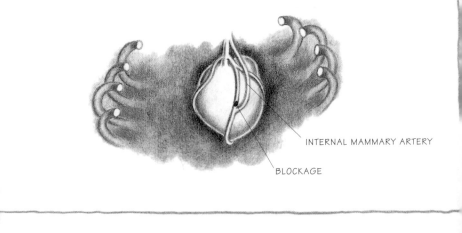

INTERNAL MAMMARY ARTERY

BLOCKAGE

What about 'after care' from a heart attack, bypass surgery, or angioplasty?

Your doctor will manage your care very closely. Generally, the cardiologist may recommend that you:
- quit smoking
- take a beta blocker drug (after a heart attack)
- lower your LDL-cholesterol below 100 mg/dL
- take a daily enteric-coated aspirin (81 mg or greater) unless you have other medical complications
- follow a "heart-healthy diet" and begin a basic exercise program, mainly walking. Always follow your doctor's recommendations.

What can be done to reduce your chances of developing heart disease?

Generally, cardiovascular disease takes a long time to develop. You may reduce your chances of developing heart disease by changing certain habits or "risk factors."

Risk factors

The primary risk factors for cardiovascular disease include:

1) Elevated cholesterol
2) Smoking
3) Diabetes
4) Hypertension
5) Obesity
6) Lack of estrogen
7) Age
8) Family history
9) Physical inactivity

1. Elevated cholesterol

Cholesterol is a "waxlike substance" that serves as a "building block" within the **cell membrane**.

CELL MEMBRANE

CHOLESTEROL

TESTOSTERONE

BILE ACID

ESTROGEN

Cholesterol is also used to make **hormones,** especially those found in reproduction: **estrogen** and **testosterone.**

Cholesterol is used to make **bile acids** that help break down fat in our intestines.

As mentioned, cholesterol may contribute to the buildup of plaque in the artery wall. Plaque restricts the flow of blood through the artery, similar to orange construction barrels you have seen on the highway. Plaque reduces the flow of blood (traffic) and increases pressure in the artery (construction zone).

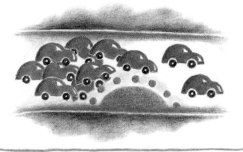

What should my cholesterol levels be?

For those individuals with coronary heart disease or diabetes, **LDL-cholesterol** should be **less than 100 mg/dL**. For individuals with two or more risk factors for cardiovascular disease, **LDL-cholesterol** should be **less than 130 mg/dL**.

Triglycerides should be **less than 200 mg/dL**.

HDL-cholesterol should be **greater than 40 mg/dL** for men and **more than 45 mg/dL** for women.

2. What about smoking?

Don't do it. Smoking is bad for the entire cardiovascular system because it:

A) Introduces carbon monoxide into the body
B) Lowers the "good" HDL-cholesterol

A. Carbon monoxide

Oxygen attaches to the red blood cells in the lungs. Red blood cells transport the oxygen throughout the body.

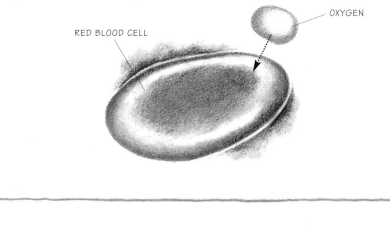

RED BLOOD CELL

OXYGEN

When you smoke, you inhale carbon monoxide into your lungs. Carbon monoxide binds to the red blood cells at the site where oxygen normally binds.

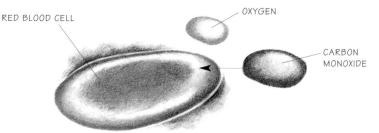

RED BLOOD CELL

OXYGEN

CARBON MONOXIDE

Therefore, less oxygen is carried by the blood, resulting in less oxygen available for use in the heart, muscles, and throughout the body. People who smoke may have abnormal heartbeats as well.

Understandably, smoking has harmful effects, especially for anyone who has already had a heart attack or bypass surgery. More importantly, there is an increased likelihood of a second heart attack or need for another bypass surgery if you continue to smoke after an initial cardiac incident.

Smoking is also a risk factor for peripheral vascular disease (blockages of the arteries to the brain, kidneys and legs).

B. Lower HDL-cholesterol

Two other reasons for
not smoking are that
it reduces the amount
of HDL-cholesterol or
"good cholesterol" in your
bloodstream, and it makes
your blood clot more easily,
increasing the potential
for an arterial blockage
(heart attack or stroke).

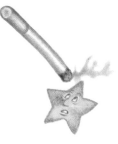

SMOKING
REDUCES
HDL-CHOLESTEROL

3. Diabetes

What exactly is diabetes? The working cells need sugar for energy. Sugar is absorbed through the digestive system after a meal or snack. **Insulin** is released by the **pancreas** to allow the body to use sugar as a source of nutrition and energy. That may be hard to visualize. This may help ...

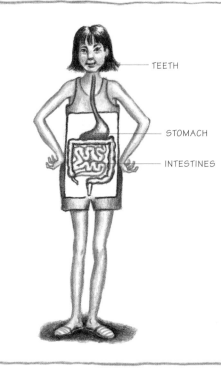

TEETH

STOMACH

INTESTINES

While you eat, the digestive system (teeth, stomach, and intestines) breaks your food down into smaller particles that are used by your body.

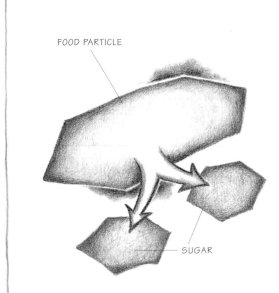

FOOD PARTICLE

SUGAR

Some food is broken down into particles of **sugar**. Sometimes this sugar is referred to as **carbohydrates** or **glucose**.

Sugar moves from the digestive system to the blood and travels throughout the body to feed the working cells. The sugar is the energy packet the cells need to do work like running and breathing.

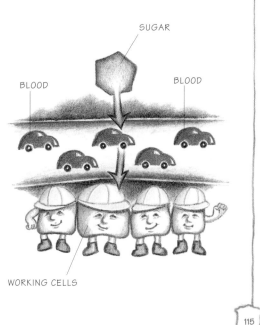

SUGAR

BLOOD

BLOOD

WORKING CELLS

At the same time, the body sends a signal to the **pancreas** telling it to release **insulin** into the bloodstream.

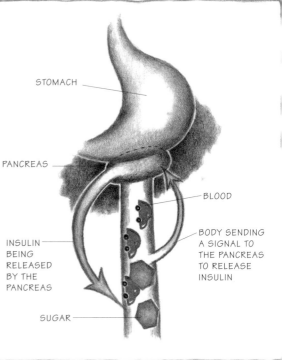

STOMACH

PANCREAS

INSULIN BEING RELEASED BY THE PANCREAS

BLOOD

BODY SENDING A SIGNAL TO THE PANCREAS TO RELEASE INSULIN

SUGAR

Insulin acts like a **key** that unlocks the doors of the cells to let sugar move in. The working cells can then use the sugar for energy to do their jobs. This is how your body uses sugar. However ...

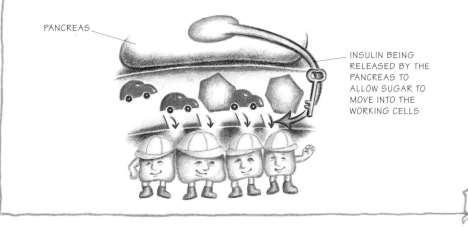

PANCREAS

INSULIN BEING RELEASED BY THE PANCREAS TO ALLOW SUGAR TO MOVE INTO THE WORKING CELLS

Without the key (insulin), the sugar cannot get out of the bloodstream and into the working cells. The sugar builds up in the blood, and the working cells get hungry. This is what happens in diabetes. A diabetic's body cannot move sugar from the blood into the cells.

Diabetes is a major risk factor for cardiovascular disease. Women over age 45 are twice as likely as men to develop diabetes. If you believe you may be at risk for diabetes, you should consult your doctor about having a simple blood glucose test.

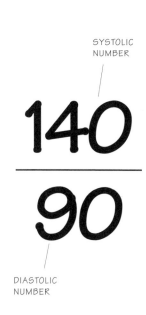

140
—
90

4. Hypertension

Hypertension is commonly referred to as high blood pressure. If you have a **systolic pressure** greater than 140 mm Hg and/or a **diastolic pressure** greater than 90 mm Hg on 2 separate visits to the doctor, then you may have high blood pressure.

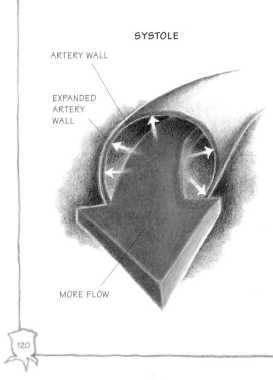

SYSTOLE

ARTERY WALL

EXPANDED ARTERY WALL

MORE FLOW

What is **systolic pressure**? Blood comes out of the heart in 1 big thrust. The artery expands to handle the blood. The amount of pressure put on the expanded artery wall is called **systolic pressure**.

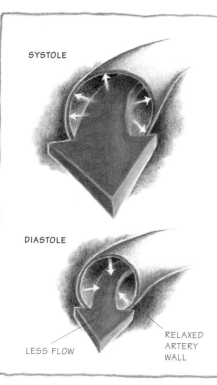

SYSTOLE

DIASTOLE

LESS FLOW

RELAXED
ARTERY
WALL

After the artery expands during systole, it relaxes back to its normal size. It is similar to a rubber band that goes back to its normal shape after being stretched. Normal pressure on the artery wall during relaxation is called **diastolic pressure**.

How does hypertension relate to cardiovascular disease?

Blood pressure is a result of the blood flowing through the artery (cardiac output) and the resistance of the artery wall (vascular resistance). If that sounds too technical, here … this may help:

Blood pressure = Cardiac output x vascular resistance

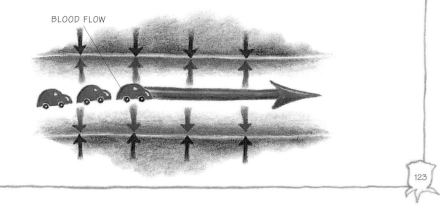

BLOOD FLOW

If a lot of resistance is created by either the blood or the artery wall, then there is more pressure as the blood travels through the artery. If it takes more energy to get the blood through the arteries, then your heart has to work harder with each beat. Most people with high blood pressure do not realize they have it. No wonder hypertension is called the "silent killer."

What contributes to hypertension?

Several factors may contribute to hypertension and cardiovascular disease. These include:

Excess dietary salt

Excess alcohol intake

Stress

Age

Genetics and family history

Obesity

Physical inactivity

High saturated fat diet

Salt

Salt helps conserve water in your body. The American Heart Association Step II Diet recommends that the average person consume no more than 2,400 mg of salt per day, especially those individuals who are salt sensitive. Excess dietary salt may contribute to both hypertension and to your body retaining too much water.

If you are retaining too much water, then you are increasing your blood volume (cars) without adding space. This increase will result in more pressure in the arteries.

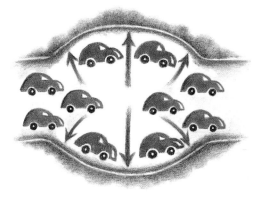

Alcohol consumption

A common concern for individuals with cardiovascular disease is alcohol consumption — mainly because there seems to be conflicting evidence about the benefits versus the risks of drinking. Experts agree that excess alcohol consumption over time can lead to many harmful effects, including high blood pressure, cirrhosis of the liver, and damage to the heart. The issue is the balance between **moderate** and **excessive** alcohol consumption. While the evidence shows that there is a protective effect for moderate alcohol consumption, this benefit disappears with excessive intake. Women should not consume more than 1 drink* each day. The 7 allowable drinks in a week should not be consumed in a few days or during a weekend of binge drinking. People who should not drink include individuals with high levels of triglycerides (over 300 mg/dL), women who are pregnant, individuals who are under age, people with a genetic predisposition for alcoholism or who are recovering alcoholics, and those taking certain medications.

*A guide: One drink is defined as 5 ounces of wine, 12 ounces of beer, or 1-1/2 ounces of 80-proof liquor.

What about stress?

When you are under stress, your brain releases signals to the body through the nerves. These signals allow your body to respond to various situations.

Arteries have nerves attached to them. The nerves can either cause the arteries to relax or can put more tension on the walls of the arteries. If you are under a lot of stress, the nerves send signals to tighten or narrow the arteries.

Narrowing the artery is like taking away a lane of traffic. There is still the same number of cars (blood) with less space (artery). This increases the pressure inside the artery.

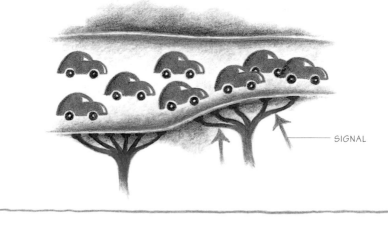

SIGNAL

So,

something you can do to improve your blood pressure is reduce stress. You can accomplish this by practicing meditation, doing deep breathing exercises, or doing exercise, such as going for a walk, riding a bike, or taking a swim.

YOGA

5. Obesity

The American Heart Association has described obesity as a major risk factor for cardiovascular disease. What exactly is obesity?

Metropolitan Life's height/weight tables are often used to determine a recommended weight for an individual based on age and gender. Generally, those who are 20% over the recommended weight for their height are considered to be overweight — but not necessarily obese. Obesity refers to fatness rather than weight. Women who have greater than 35% of their body weight as fat are considered to be obese. Obesity and being overweight carry significant health risks, are directly related to cardiovascular risk factors, and may:

1) raise triglycerides (a "bad" blood fat)
2) lower HDL-cholesterol (the "good" cholesterol)
3) raise LDL-cholesterol (the "bad" cholesterol)
4) raise blood pressure and
5) increase the risk of developing diabetes

Obesity may be related to both genetics (nature) and lifestyle (nurture). Generally speaking, obesity occurs when the calories we consume exceed the calories we burn through activities of daily living and exercise. We store the excess calories as fat reserves, thus contributing to obesity and ultimately increasing the risk of coronary disease. Obesity has increased in women in every decade over the past 50 years. There is a misconception that Americans are overeating and eating too much fat. In fact, as a nation we are eating less fat, fewer calories, and still gaining weight — primarily due to the lower levels of physical activity in our youth and adult lives. A sedentary lifestyle could be the real culprit.

6. Lack of estrogen

The most common cause of death in women and men is cardiovascular disease. Women and men share the same risk factors for heart disease.

Women, throughout the years they experience a menstrual cycle, have the benefit of circulating estrogen. Estrogen is mainly produced by the ovaries.

Estrogen may protect women from heart disease by increasing **HDL-cholesterol** ("good cholesterol") and by having special effects on the walls of blood vessels.

When women reach menopause, their ovaries lose the ability to produce estrogen. At this time, there is an increase in the number of women who develop coronary heart disease. Coronary heart disease occurs in 1 out of 3 women after age 65.

There is a way to replace some of the lost estrogen in a postmenopausal woman.

How can estrogen be replaced?

Estrogen can be replaced through medication known as **hormone replacement therapy** or **HRT**. HRT includes 2 hormones: **estrogen** and **progesterone**. Many studies show that women who take these hormones could reduce their risk of coronary heart disease by up to 50%. The main benefit is seen with **estrogen**.

Estrogen's benefits in hormone replacement may work through the following ways:

1) Lowering **total cholesterol** and increasing the **HDL-cholesterol** ("good" cholesterol)
2) Increasing the size of the openings of heart arteries for blood flow
3) Preventing plaque formation in the arteries

Progesterone, another hormone, is taken with estrogen to protect the lining of the uterus against endometrial cancer. This does not apply to women who do not have a uterus because of a **hysterectomy**. Progesterone can impact the benefits of estrogen, depending on the type of progesterone prescribed by your doctor.

Other benefits of HRT include reducing the risk of osteoporosis and improving menopausal symptoms. Complications of HRT can include increased risk of breast cancer, increased rates of blood clots in the deep veins, and stroke. Some side effects include irregular bleeding, bloating, and breast tenderness.

There are many ways that HRT can be prescribed by your doctor. **You must talk to your doctor before taking hormones or any other medications. Be sure that you are able to take estrogen and/or progesterone. Certain medical conditions may prohibit you from taking HRT. Your doctor can discuss all the risks and benefits of HRT.**

7. Age

Aging has an effect on the risk of cardiovascular disease because aging causes changes in the heart and blood vessels. As people age, they become less active, gain more weight, and the effects of a sedentary lifestyle, smoking, and poor diet continue to damage the heart and circulation by increasing blood pressure and cholesterol levels. Blood pressure increases with aging, in part because arteries gradually lose some of their elasticity and, over time, may not be as resilient.

8. Family history

A **family history** of cardiovascular disease could reflect genetics and/or an unhealthy family lifestyle. If most of your family members smoke, are sedentary, and have a poor diet — then these are harmful habits that increase the risk of heart disease in your family. However, unlike your genes, these behaviors can be changed.

On the other hand, if your family has a healthful lifestyle but there is still a high incidence of cardiovascular disease, then it is likely that genetics is playing a role. We are learning more about the importance of genetic risk for vascular disease. In the future, treatment may be tailored to an individual's own genetic makeup. In either case, by practicing a healthful lifestyle, you can help reduce your risk rather than giving up and thinking you have no control over your destiny.

9. Physical inactivity

Lack of exercise is a major contributor to obesity, diabetes, and hypertension. Beginning an exercise program may help you feel better, help you have more energy, help you lose some weight, lower your cholesterol, lower your blood pressure, help you look better, and improve your muscle tone. Also, beginning an exercise routine can increase your HDL-cholesterol or "good cholesterol" — especially if exercise is associated with weight loss.

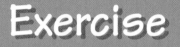

Currently, only 22% of adults in the United States exercise at a level that benefits their cardiovascular systems. What are some important considerations?

1) Type of exercise

2) Amount and regularity of exercise

3) Intensity of exercise

1. Type of exercise

Aerobic exercise

To meet your general fitness goals, the best type of exercise is **aerobic** exercise.

Aerobic exercise does not necessarily require special equipment or a health club membership. Aerobic exercises are those that require a lot of oxygen. These exercises include walking, jogging, cycling, swimming, cross-country skiing, or rowing.

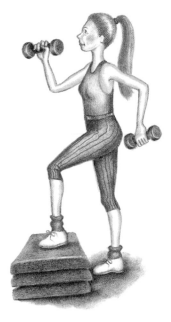

20-30 minutes a day, 5 days a week

2. Amount and regularity of exercise

The U.S. surgeon general recommends that healthy adults exercise 20 to 30 minutes, 5 days a week.

There are nearly 50 half hours in a 24-hour day. Exercising for 30 minutes daily requires **only about 2%** of your total day. Try to find 1, or 2, or 3 exercises you like to do. You'll enjoy the variety.

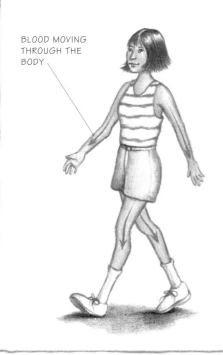

BLOOD MOVING THROUGH THE BODY

3. Intensity of exercise

Warm up

By walking or cycling slowly, you move the blood out to the working muscles. A warm-up should start slowly and last 5 to 10 minutes.

You cannot maintain "all out" exercise (100%) for very long. An example of an "all out" exercise is sprinting. Actually, you may only maintain a sprint for about 15 seconds.

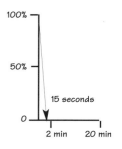

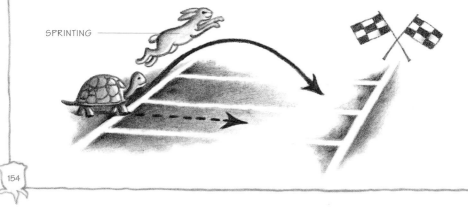

SPRINTING

If you slow the exercise down a bit, to about 90%, you may still only go for about 2 minutes!

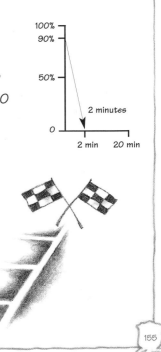

What if you slow your exercise down to 75% or even 50%? There is a **huge** difference. Now you may easily go more than 20 minutes.

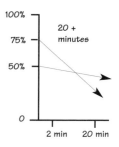

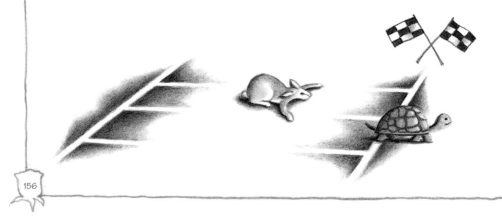

Simply —

By slowing down the pace, you may be able to exercise for a longer period of time.

Many exercise physiologists use the following generally accepted formula to determine the exercise target heart rate of a healthy individual. If you have a history of cardiovascular disease, or if you are just starting a program, **check with your doctor before starting an exercise routine**. Your doctor is aware of the many factors that may need to be considered in modifying your exercise intensity.

Target heart rate example

Your age: 50

1. 220 minus your age:
2. Answer #1 minus
   your resting pulse:
3. Answer #2 times 0.5:
4. Answer #3 plus
   your resting pulse:
5. Answer #2 times 0.75:
6. Answer #5 plus
   your resting pulse:
7. **Target heart rate** equals
   range between values for
   #4 and #6:

Your resting pulse: 70

1. 220 - 50 = 170

2. 170 - 70 = 100
3. 100 x 0.5 = 50

4. 50 + 70 = 120

5. 100 x 0.75 = 75

6. 75 + 70 = 145

7. **120 to 145 beats
   per minute, or 12 to 14
   beats for 6 seconds**

Now it's your turn

Here is how you determine the heart rate of an apparently healthy individual. Please consult with your doctor to make sure that this is an accurate target heart rate for your condition.

1. Measure your pulse (heart rate) for 60 seconds: _____
2. Take 220 and subtract your age: 220 - _____ = _____
3. Now take the answer in #2 and subtract your pulse: _____
4. Take the answer in #3 and multiply by 0.5: _____
5. Take the answer in #4 and add your pulse: _____
6. Take the answer in #3 and multiply by 0.75: _____
7. Take the answer in #6 and add your pulse: _____
8. Your target heart rate should range from the answer in #5 (_____) to the answer in #7 (_____).
9. Divide each answer in #8 by 10 to determine your pulse for 6 seconds: _____ to _____.

How hard and how often should I exercise?

When you are just starting out, try to exercise very comfortably. Here are 4 quick tips.

1) Try to exercise so that you are breathing noticeably but are **not** out of breath. Remember this simple rule: you should be able to carry on a conversation while you are exercising.

2) Sweating is a good thing. This means that your body is working hard enough and receiving the necessary stimulus for the muscles and the heart.

3) If you are not fatigued and are completely recovered from exercising on the previous day, then you should exercise **daily**.

4) Give yourself a **warm-up** before exercise (several minutes of easy walking) and a **cooldown** at the end of exercise (again, several minutes of easy walking). Ask an exercise specialist for some recommendations for stretching after your workout, and discuss the intensity of the exercise with your doctor.

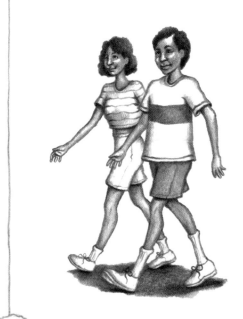

If you are just starting an exercise program, probably the simplest exercise to try is walking. It is fairly easy to do for 20 minutes. Check with your doctor for any additional input on your exercise program.

VERY, VERY important

Cool down. As important as the warm-up and the aerobic exercise are to improving your fitness, you must also include a cooldown as part of your exercise routine.

Your cooldown should be just like your warm-up. At the end of your exercise routine, give yourself 5 to 10 minutes of nice, easy walking. You also may want to include some mild stretching.

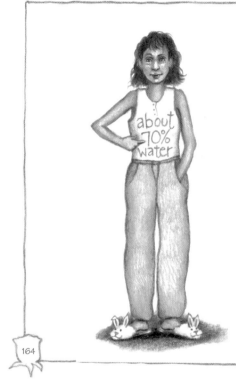

Another consideration — water

Water is needed for virtually every function of the body. The body is approximately 70% water.

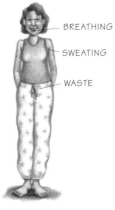

BREATHING
SWEATING
WASTE

During the course of the day, you lose water through sweating, breathing, and waste. Replacement of water (rehydration) is important — especially when participating in an exercise program.

A prudent recommendation is that you should drink 6 to 10 glasses of water per day. Sorry, caffeinated drinks and alcohol do not count. They are "diuretics," meaning that they actually may cause you to lose even more water.

Questions

Here are some questions
that you may want to take
with you the next time you
go to see your doctor.

What are my medications? How does each of them help me?

Answer _____

_____

_____

_____

_____

_____

_____

_____

List the blood pressure reading for each visit to your doctor and the date.

Date	Blood pressure
_____	_____
_____	_____
_____	_____
_____	_____
_____	_____
_____	_____

Do I have any exercise limitations of which I should be aware? What are they?

Answer _____

_____

Should I have a treadmill test before I start to exercise? What is my target heart rate?

Answer _____

_____

Based on my weight, blood pressure, and blood cholesterol level, should I talk to someone about changing my diet?

Yes   No

Contact your local hospital for the name of a registered dietitian.

Dietitian _____

Address _____

_____

Phone _____

If I have heart disease, are there any concerns that I should be aware of before having/resuming sexual activity?

Answer _____

_____

_____

_____

Am I a candidate for HRT?

Answer _____

_____

Do I need to get a mammogram? How often?

Answer _____

_____

Do I need to get a DEXA scan?

Answer _____

_____

What can I change in my diet and exercise routine to help me with osteoporosis?

Answer _____

_____

What treatment is best for me if I have osteoporosis?

Answer _____

_____

What treatment is best for me if I have breast cancer?

Answer _____

_____

_____

_____

_____

Woman to Woman …

We hope that this book has increased your understanding about breast cancer, osteoporosis, and heart disease. We cannot stress enough how vital it is to consult with your doctor about risks, prevention, and treatment of these diseases. We hope that you will be able to take steps in your life to help reduce your chance of developing breast cancer, osteoporosis, and heart disease. If you happen to have one of these illnesses, we want you to know there are treatments your doctor can offer you. You should also be able to ask your doctor questions about health issues specific to you. Please remember, take the time to take care of yourself. You are a very special woman!

Bibliography

American Cancer Society on breast cancer at http://www3.cancer.org accessed February 1999.

American Cancer Society Recommendations Screening Mammogram. Facts and Figures. July 1998.

American College of Obstetrics and Gynecology Technical Bulletin. "Hormone Replacement Therapy." April 1992: 166.

American College of Sports Medicine position stand. "The Recommended Quality and Quantity of Exercise for Developing and Maintaining Cardiorespiratory and Muscular Fitness in Healthy Adults." *Medicine and Science in Sports and Exercise* April 1990.

American Heart Association consensus panel statement. "Preventing Heart Attack and Death in Patients With Coronary Disease." *Circulation* 1995; 2-4.

The American Journal of Managed Care Special Report. Creating an Optimal Strategy of Treating Endometriosis and Chronic Pelvic Pain. May 1999. Volume 5. Number 5. Suppl.

Angell, M. "Caring for women's health – what is the problem?" *New England Journal of Medicine* 1993: 271.

Association of Professors of Obstetrics and Gynecology Educational Series on Women's Health Issues. "Osteoporosis, Treatment, Monitoring." 1996.

Baker, V.D., and R.B. Jaffe. "Clinical uses of antiestrogens." *Obstetric Gynecological Survey* Jan. 1995: 45-49.

Burke, A.P., and A. Farb, G.T. Malcom, Y. Liang, J. Smialek, R. Virmani. "Coronary Risk Factors and Plaque Morphology in Men with Coronary Disease Who Died Suddenly." *New England Journal of Medicine* 1 May 1997: 1276-1282.

Cogswell, M.E. "Nicotine Withdrawal Symptoms." *North Carolina Medical Journal* 1 Jan. 1995: 40-45.

Collins, R., and R. Peto, C. Baigent, P. Sleight. "Aspirin, Heparin, and Fibrinolytic Therapy in Suspected Acute Myocardial Infarction." *New England Journal of Medicine* 20 March 1997: 847-860.

Cummings, S., and M.C. Nevitt, W.S. Browner, K. Stone, K.M. Fox, K.E. Ensrud, J. Cauley, D. Black, T.M. Vogt for The Study of Osteoporotic Fractures Research Group. "Risk factors for hip fractures in white women." *New England Journal of Medicine* 23 March 1995.

Da Costa, F.D., et al. "Myocardial Revascularization with the Radial Artery: A Clinical and Angiographic Study." *Annals of Thoracic Surgery* Aug. 1996: 475-480.

Delmas, P.D., et al. "Effects of raloxifene on bone mineral density, serum cholesterol concentrations, and uterine endometrium in postmenopausal women." *New England Journal of Medicine* 4 Dec. 1997: 1641-1647.

Eckel, R.H. "Obesity in Heart Disease." *Circulation* 1997: 3248-3250.

Executive Summary of the Third Report of the National Cholesterol Education Program (NCEP) Expert Panel on Detection, Evaluation, and Treatment of High Blood Cholesterol in Adults (Adult Treatment Panel III). JAMA, May 16, 2001, Vol. 285, No. 19: 2486-2497.

Fernando, G.R., R.M. Martha, and R. Evangelina. "Consumption of soft drinks with phosphoric acid as a risk factor for the development of hypocalcemia in postmenopausal women." *Journal of Clinical Epidemiology* Oct. 1999: 1007-1010.

Fisher, B., et al. "Tamoxifen for Prevention of Breast Cancer: Report of the National Surgical Adjuvant Breast and Bowel Project P-1 Study." *Journal of the National Cancer Institute,* Sept. 1998: 572-578; 1371-1388.

Friedman, G.D., and A.L. Klatsky. "Is Alcohol Good for Your Health?" *New England Journal of Medicine* 16 Dec. 1993: 1882-1883.

Gartside, P.S., P. Wang, and C.J. Glueck. "Prospective assessment of coronary heart disease risk factors: The NHANES I Epidemiologic Follow-up Study (HNEFS) 16 follow up." *Journal of the American College of Nutrition.* 1999; 17: 263-269.

Gellar, A. "Common Addictions." *Clinical Symposia.* Ciba-Geigy Corporation. 1996.

Grossman, E., and F.H. Messerli. "Diabetic and Hypertensive Heart Disease." *Annals of Internal Medicine* 15 Aug. 1996: 304-310.

Harris, J.R., M.E. Lipman, M. Morrow, and S. Helman. Diseases of the Breast. Philadelphia: Lippencott and Raven. 1996.

Heaney, R.P. "Calcium — answers for lifelong health." Supplement to OBG Management. Dec. 1998.

Heaney, R.P. "Pathophysiology of Osteoporosis." *Endocrinology Metabolism Clinics of North America* 27 June 1998: 255-265.

Henningfield, J.D., and R.M. Keenan. "The Anatomy of Nicotine Addiction." *Health Values* March/April 1993: 12-19.

Hutchings, O., et al. "Effect of early American results on patients in a Tamoxifen prevention trial." *Lancet* 10 Oct. 1998: 1222.

Joint National Committee. The Fifth Report of the Joint National Committee on Detection, Evaluation, and Treatment of High Blood Pressure. Bethesda (MD): National Institutes of Health, National Heart, Lung, and Blood Institute; 1993. NIH publication No. 93-1008.

Kannel, W.B., and R.B. D'Agostino, J.L. Cobb. "Effects of Weight on Cardiovascular Disease." *American Journal of Clinical Nutrition* March 1996: 419S-422S.

Kenney, W.L., et al. *American College of Sports Medicine Guidelines for Exercise Testing and Prescription.* 5th ed. Media, Pa.: Williams & Wilkins, 1995.

Margolis, S., and P.J. Goldschmidt-Clermont. *The Johns-Hopkins White Papers.* Baltimore: The Johns-Hopkins Medical Institutions, 1996.

Massey, L.K. "Caffeine and the elderly." *Drugs and Aging* July 1998: 43-50.

McCarron, D.A., and M.E. Reusser. "Body Weight and Blood Pressure Regulation." *American Journal of Clinical Nutrition* March 1996: 423S-425S.

The Medical Letter. "Raloxifene for postmenopausal osteoporosis." Vol. 40 (Issue 1022), 13 March 1998.

Meeker, M.H., and J.C. Rothrock. *Alexander's Care of the Patient in Surgery,* 10th ed. St. Louis: Mosby, 1995.

National Cancer Institute on breast cancer at http://www.nci.nih.gov accessed March 1999.

National Institutes of Health Consensus Development Conference Statement on Osteoporosis at http://www.osteo.org accessed March 1999.

Peterson, J.A., and C.X. Bryant. *The Fitness Handbook;* 2nd ed. St. Louis: Wellness Bookshelf, 1995.

Prestwood, K.M., and A.M. Kenny. "Osteoporosis: pathogenesis, diagnosis, and treatment in older adults." *Clinics in Geriatric Medicine.* 14 Aug. 1998: 577-599.

Ryan, T.J., and J.L. Anderson, E.M. Autman, et al. "ACC/AHA Guidelines for the Management of Patients with Acute Myocardial Infarction: A Report of the American College of Cardiology/American Heart Association Task Force on Practice Guidelines (Committee on Management of Acute Myocardial Infarction)." *Journal of the American College of Cardiology* 1 Nov. 1996: 1328-1428.

St. Jeor, S.T., and K.D. Brownell, R.L. Atkinson, C. Bouchard, et al. "Obesity Workshop III." *Circulation* 1996: 1391-1396.

Scheiber, L.B., and L. Torregrosa. "Early intervention for postmenopausal osteoporosis." *Journal of Musculoskeletal Medicine* March 1999: 146-157.

Scheiber, L.B., and L. Torregrosa. "Early intervention for postmenopausal osteoporosis." *Journal of Musculoskeletal Medicine* May 1999: 276-285.

Schlant, R.C., and R.W. Alexander. *The Heart*, 8th ed. New York: McGraw-Hill, 1994.

Spense, A., and M. Elliot. Human Anatomy and Physiology, 3rd Ed. California: Benjamin/Cummings Publishing Company Inc., 1987.

Speroff, L., R. Glass, and N. Kase. Clinical Gynecologic Endocrinology and Infertility, 5th Ed. Williams and Wilkins, 1994.

Superko, H.R. "The Most Common Cause of Coronary Heart Disease can be Successfully Treated by the Least Expensive Therapy — Exercise." *Certified News* 1998: 1-5.

United States Department of Health and Human Services, NIH, NIA. "Osteoporosis: The Silent Bone Thinner." 1996.

United States Surgeon General on his priorities at http://www.osophs.dhhs.gov/myjob/priorities.htm accessed November 1999.

Voors, A.A., et al. "Smoking and Cardiac Events After Venous Coronary Bypass Surgery." *Circulation* Jan. 1, 1995: 42-47.

Voutilainen, S., et al. "Angiographic 5-Year Follow-up Study of Right Gastroepiploic Artery Grafts." *Annals of Thoracic Surgery* Aug. 1996: 501-505.

Wenger, N.K. "Coronary heart disease: an older woman's major health risk." *British Medical Journal* 25 Oct. 1997: 1085-1090.

White H.D., and J.J. Van de Werf. "Thrombolysis for Acute Myocardial Infarction." *Circulation* 28 April 1998: 1632-1646.

Zelasko, C.J. "Exercise for Weight Loss: What Are the Facts?" *Journal of the American Dietetic Association* Dec. 1995: 973-1031.

About the Authors

Caroline J. Böhme, MD, FACOG, is an Obstetrician and Gynecologist for the Crescent Women's Medical Group as well as Staff Physician in Obstetrics and Gynecology at Bethesda Hospital. She lives in Cincinnati, Ohio.

Janette Gosch-Weisbrodt, MEd, is Strength and Conditioning Coordinator at a large Midwest manufacturing company. She lives in Cincinnati, Ohio.

Rona B. Wharton, MEd, RD, LD, is Clinical Nutrition Manager for the Carolinas Hospital System. She lives in Florence, South Carolina.
